SPREADING
the
WORD
G*of*OD

A GUIDE FOR RELIGIOUS
EXEMPTION TO IMMUNIZATION
WITH BIBLICAL SCRIPTURE REFERENCE

Tiffany Guay

ISBN 978-1-0980-2848-0 (paperback)
ISBN 978-1-0980-2849-7 (digital)

Christian Faith Publishing, Inc.
832 Park Avenue
Meadville, PA 16335
www.christianfaithpublishing.com

Unless otherwise indicated, Scripture quotations are from the Holy Bible, New International Version, copyright 2008-2019. Life Church Scripture quotations identified NIV are from the New International Version.

Printed in the United States of America

Say to him: Long life to you! Good health to you
and your household! And good health to all that is yours!

—1 Samuel 25:6

ACKNOWLEDGMENTS

I want to thank my queen mother for many things, such as always encouraging me in all of my endeavors. She taught me all she knows about vitamins and grocery shopping.

She always believed in me. She was my taxi driver to and from my volunteer job at the Osteopathic Community General Hospital. She encouraged me to pursue a high school internship at a chiropractic office. She called me her Gypsy Wanderer. Thanks to travel, I have learned perspective and gained experience. And finally, I want to thank my queen mother for encouraging me to expand my humble report into a book that could help many.

I want to thank my dad for giving me many gifts of true life value. Not only did my dad train me to be a strong, resilient athlete that fights the good fight. But he also developed in me a deep love and need for reading books—a need to learn all that I can. Books can be an adventure. Books can fuel ones thirst for knowledge. So thank you, Dad, for the great example of looking in a book, searching for the truth, thinking for myself, rising above, and carrying on joyfully.

I want to thank my husband, of course. He has stood beside me for a solid twenty years. He has endured my hot topic discussions on PETA, veganism/vegetarianism, holistic health and wellness, religion, and politics. I do repay the kindness by enduring sports center debates and fantasy football smack talk. That's love! I thank you immensely for having the trust and faith in me to guide you and our family and friends toward optimal life choices in the health avenue.

I want to thank my dear, sweet, little boy, who I cherish so much. He fills me with passion and love. Because I have him to protect, I have gained much wisdom. I have been filled up, to the point of overflowing.

I thank the Lord, our God and Savior. He has trained me for the moment such as this.

> The Lord is my shepherd, I lack nothing. He makes me lie down in green pastures, he leads me beside quiet waters, he refreshes my soul. He guides me along the right paths for his name's sake. Even though I walk through the darkest valley, I will fear no evil, for you are with me; your rod and your staff, they comfort me. You prepare a table before me in the presence of my enemies. You anoint my head with oil; my cup overflows. Surely your goodness and love will follow me all the days of my life, and I will dwell in the house of the Lord forever. (Psalm 23)

CONTENTS

AUTHOR'S NOTES

Why did I write this book?

I wrote this book because God gave me a lifelong passion for health. I have been blessed with education, and I want to educate and inform others. In hopes of sharing the Good News of the Gospel, you will know that God made us in his image, to be like him. He is our Father in heaven. The Bible is God's instruction book on how we should live. We all want abundant good health. We want a fulfilling marriage. We want not only to have good friends and a good family, but we want to be a good friend and bring goodness to our family. We want to excel at our jobs. We want many things out of this life God gave us to enjoy. He also gave us freedom to choose to make our own decisions. That is where the good old Bible comes into play. The "playbook." Through stories and adventures of those who have come before us, God tells us all of the pathways that we can journey through this life. He makes a straight way for us to follow; we just have to follow. And when we struggle to make the best choice, we just have to pray for guidance. God does listen to our hearts' desires. And God does work all things together for his good, and the glory of his kingdom. Because he is good. So let me tell you all. As you read this book and you learn how God has instructed us to keep our bodies pure; what not to put into our bodies, how to treat other's lives (human and animal), how to treat ourselves, moral character to uphold, his commandments, all of this and more, I cover briefly by showing scripture references. Yet how much more knowledge we can gain from the good old Bible, written thousands of years ago. I encourage you to be curious, open God's Book, and take a look. You will be glad you did. I will be glad you did too. My hope is that all people that read my book will see the light of the truth.

Let God shine through you. Stand upon his Word. If you already have a relationship with God, let his words awaken you. If you have never had the opportunity to know God but you have a faith in a higher power of this universe, now's your time. Be curious.

INTRODUCTION

Letter to the Building Principal

Dear building principal,

I, your name here, the parent of your child's name here, am submitting for review, my parental statement requesting for religious exemption to immunization. Due to my sincere and genuine religious beliefs, I thank you for your time while considering my request.

Explain in your own words why you are requesting this religious exemption.

Title 77 of the Illinois Administrative Code, Chapter 1, Subchapter I, Part 665.510 gives me the right as a parent to object to my child's vaccinations on religious grounds.

I am objecting to vaccines because I believe in and follow God and the principles laid out in his Word, and I deeply believe that vaccines violate them.

Describe the religious principles that guide your objection to immunization.

At least twenty-seven vaccines contain cells, cellular debris, protein, and DNA from aborted babies including (but not limited to) Adenovirus, Polio, DTaP-polio-Hib combo, hepatitis A, hepatitis A-B combo, MMR, MMRV ProQuad, rabies, varicella, shingles vaccines, Ebola, HIV, tuberculosis, malaria, and influenza vaccines. (http://www.cdc.gov/vaccines/pubs/pinkbook/downloads/appe ndices/B/excipient-table-2.PDF)

(see attached: "Vaccine Excipient and Media Summary")

- "Thou shalt not murder" (Exodus 20:13, Deuteronomy 5:17).
- "Children are recognized from God at the point of conception" (Genesis 4:1, Jeremiah 1:5).
- "Children are knit together by God in the womb" (Psalm 139:13–16, Psalm 22:10–11).
- "Children are blessings from God" (Genesis 1:28, Genesis 4:1, Psalm 127:3, Psalm 113:7–9).
- "Children are valued and loved" (Matthew 18:1–14, Matthew 19:13–15).
- "Children are created in His image" (Genesis 1:27).
- "And their killing is condemned" (Psalm 106:35, 37–38).
- "The prophet Amos condemns the Ammonites because he 'ripped open expectant mothers in Gilead'" (Amos 1:13).
- "And child killing was one of the major reasons that God's anger burned against the Kingdom of Israel bringing about their destruction and exile" (2 Kings 17:17–18).
- Your body is a temple for the Holy Spirit.
- "Do you not know that your bodies are temples of the Holy Spirit, who is in you, whom you have received from God? You are not your own; you were bought at a price. Therefore honor God with your bodies" (1 Corinthians 6:19–20).

Vaccines contain neurotoxins, hazardous substances, attenuated viruses, animal parts, foreign DNA, albumin from human blood, carcinogens, and chemical wastes that are proven harmful to the human body.

Not only are the additives in vaccines considered contaminants from a biblical standpoint; the contaminants themselves are often contaminated.

In the Bible, blood represented the life force of the human or animal. Human blood was to be kept pure under all circumstances and free of contaminants like animal parts and blood (Genesis 9:4; Leviticus 17:10–11, 17:14; Deuteronomy 12:23; Acts 15:20, 15:29).

Since vaccine preparation involves the use of materials of biological origin, vaccines are subject to contamination by microorganisms. The increasing number of target species for vaccines, the diversity of the origin of biological materials, and the viruses and their constant evolution represent a challenge to vaccine producers and regulatory authorities (https://www.ncbI.nlm.nih.gov/pubmed/20456974) (see attached: "Human and animal vaccine contaminations").

My God is a sovereign God. It is a parent's God-given authority over the care of their children, that intentionally exposing the immuno-compromised and others to the live viral shedding that accompanies vaccines or subjecting your child to a risk of chronic disease and even death violates the command to love your neighbor as yourself.

> "God prohibits child sacrifice" (Exodus 20:13, Deuteronomy 5:17, 12:30–32, 18:10; 2 Kings 16:2–3; Psalm 106:38; Leviticus 18:21, 20:1–5).

I read and follow God's Word:

> "Trust in the Lord with all of your heart and do not lean on your own understanding. In all your ways acknowledge Him, and He will make your paths straight" (Proverbs 3:5–6).

The Bible does not reference vaccines specifically, but it does reference pharmaceuticals, to which vaccines belong. You know what the Bible calls this? Sorcery. Actually, the Greek word for sorcery is *pharmakeia*. (Galatians 5:14–21; Revelations 9:21, 18:23, 21:8, 22:15–16).

Indicate whether you are opposed to all immunizations and, if not, the religious basis that prohibits particular immunizations.

I am opposed to all vaccinations.

(https://www.livingwhole.org/resources/)

Sincerely,
Your name here

Dear readers,

I love our country, and I am a very proud citizen. I am a wife and mother. I am a certified natural chef and natural health consultant. I am a small business owner. I am a hard worker, and I appreciate all people and our individual uniqueness. I volunteer in children's ministry. I grew up always learning and trying my best, to follow the way our Lord teaches us in his book, the Bible. I celebrate life as an American. I will honor and protect all of our freedoms that this country has worked hard on founding.

> The First Amendment of the United States Constitution protects the right to freedom of religion and freedom of expression from government interference. It prohibits any laws that establish a national religion, impede the free exercise of religion, abridge the freedom of speech, infringe upon the freedom of the press, interfere with the right to peaceably assemble, or prohibit citizens from petitioning for a governmental redress of grievances. (*First Amendment: An Overview*, Cornell Law School)

It was adopted into the Bill of Rights in 1791.

I would love to share with you what it means to me to have a religious exemption from immunization. My book shows references in the Bible that supports our need for religious exemption from immunization. In God we trust.

Sincerely,
Thank you for hearing me,
Tiffany A. T. Guay

VACCINE EXCIPIENT
AND MEDIA SUMMARY

Excipients Included in U.S. Vaccines, by Vaccine

In addition to weakened or killed disease antigens (viruses or bacteria), vaccines contain very small amounts of other ingredients—excipients or media.

Some excipients are added to a vaccine for a specific purpose. These include:

Preservatives, to prevent contamination. For example, thimerosal.

Adjuvants, to help stimulate a stronger immune response. For example, aluminum salts.

Stabilizers, to keep the vaccine potent during transportation and storage. For example, sugars or gelatin.

Others are residual trace amounts of materials that were used during the manufacturing process and removed. These include:

Cell culture materials, used to grow the vaccine antigens. For example, egg protein, various culture media. Inactivating ingredients, used to kill viruses or inactivate toxins. For example, formaldehyde. Antibiotics, used to prevent contamination by bacteria. For example, neomycin.

The following table lists all components, other than antigens, shown in the manufacturers' package insert (PI) for each vaccine. Each of these PIs, which can be found on the FDA's website (see below) contains a description of that vaccine's manufacturing process, including the amount and purpose of each substance. In most PIs, this information is found in Section 11: "Description."

All information was extracted from manufacturers' package inserts.

If in doubt about whether a PI has been updated since this table was prepared, check the FDA's website at:
http://www.fda.gov/BiologicsBloodVaccines/Vaccines/ApprovedProducts/ucm093833.htm

Vaccine	Contains
Adenovirus	Human-diploid fibroblast cell cultures (strain WI-38), Dulbecco's Modified Eagle's Medium, fetal bovine serum, sodium bicarbonate, monosodium glutamate, sucrose, D-mannose, D-fructose, dextrose, human serum albumin, potassium phosphate, plasdone C, anhydrous lactose, microcrystalline cellulose, polacrilin potassium, magnesium stearate, cellulose acetate phthalate, alcohol, acetone, castor oil, FD&C Yellow #6 aluminum lake dye
Anthrax (Biothrax)	Amino acids, vitamins, inorganic salts, sugars, aluminum hydroxide, sodium chloride, benzethonium chloride, formaldehyde
BCG (Tice)	Glycerin, asparagine, citric acid, potassium phosphate, magnesium sulfate, iron ammonium citrate, lactose
Cholera (Vaxchora)	Casamino acids, yeast extract, mineral salts, anti-foaming agent, ascorbic acid, hydrolyzed casein, sodium chloride, sucrose, dried lactose, sodium bicarbonate, sodium carbonate
DT (Sanofi)	Aluminum phosphate, isotonic sodium chloride, formaldehyde, casein, cystine, maltose, uracil, inorganic salts, vitamins, dextrose
DTaP (Daptacel)	Aluminum phosphate, formaldehyde, glutaraldehyde, 2-phenoxyethanol, Stainer-Scholte medium, casamino acids, dimethyl-beta-cyclodextrin, Mueller's growth medium, ammonium sulfate, modified Mueller-Miller casamino acid medium without beef heart infusion
DTaP (Infanrix)	Fenton medium containing a bovine extract, modified Latham medium derived from bovine casein, formaldehyde, modified Stainer-Scholte liquid medium, glutaraldehyde, aluminum hydroxide, sodium chloride, polysorbate 80 (Tween 80)

DTaP-IPV (Kinrix)	Fenton medium containing a bovine extract, modified Latham medium derived from bovine casein, formaldehyde, modified Stainer-Scholte liquid medium, glutaraldehyde, aluminum hydroxide, VERO cells, a continuous line of monkey kidney cells, Calf serum, lactalbumin hydrolysate, sodium chloride, polysorbate 80 (Tween 80), neomycin sulfate, polymyxin B
DTaP-IPV (Quadracel)	Modified Mueller's growth medium, ammonium sulfate, modified Mueller-Miller casamino acid medium without beef heart infusion, formaldehyde, aluminum phosphate, Stainer-Scholte medium, casamino acids, dimethyl-beta-cyclodextrin, MRC-5 cells, normal human diploid cells, CMRL 1969 medium supplemented with calf serum, Medium 199 without calf serum, 2-phenoxycthanol, polysorbate 80, glutaraldehyde, neomycin, polymyxin B sulfate
DTaP-HepB-IPV (Pediarix)	Fenton medium containing a bovine extract, modified Latham medium derived from bovine casein, formaldehyde, glutaraldehyde, modified Stainer-Scholte liquid medium, VERO cells, a continuous line of monkey kidney cells, calf serum and lactalbumin hydrolysate, aluminum hydroxide, aluminum phosphate, aluminum salts, sodium chloride, polysorbate 80 (Tween 80), neomycin sulfate, polymyxin B, yeast protein.
DTaP-IPV/ Hib (Pentacel)	Aluminum phosphate, polysorbate 80, sucrose, formaldehyde, glutaraldehyde, bovine serum albumin, 2-phcnoxyethanol, neomycin, polymyxin B sulfate, modified Mueller's growth medium, ammonium sulfate, modified Mueller-Miller casamino acid medium without beef heart infusion, Stainer-Scholte medium, casamino acids, dimethyl-beta-cyclodextrin. MRC-5 cells (a line of normal human diploid cells), CMRL 1969 medium supplemented with calf serum. Medium 199 without calf serum, modified Mueller and Miller medium
Hib (ActHIB)	Sodium chloride, modified Mueller and Miller medium (the culture medium contains milk-derived raw materials [casein derivatives]), formaldehyde, sucrose
Hib (Hiberix)	Saline, synthetic medium, formaldehyde, sodium chloride, lactose
Hib (PedvaxHIB)	Complex fermentation media, amorphous aluminum hydroxyphosphate sulfate, sodium chloride
Hep A (Havrix)	MRC-5 human diploid cells, formalin, aluminum hydroxide, amino acid supplement, phosphate-buffered saline solution, polysorbate 20, neomycin sulfate, aminoglycoside antibiotic

Hep A (Vaqta)	MRC-5 diploid fibroblasts, amorphous aluminum hydroxyphosphate sulfate, non-viral protein, DNA, bovine albumin, formaldehyde, neomycin, sodium borate, sodium chloride
Hep B (Engerix-B)	Aluminum hydroxide, yeast protein, sodium chloride, disodium phosphate dihydrate, sodium dihydrogen phosphate dihydrate
Hep B (Recombivax)	Soy peptone, dextrose, amino acids, mineral salts, phosphate buffer, formaldehyde, potassium aluminum sulfate, amorphous aluminum hydroxyphosphate sulfate, yeast protein
Hep B (Heplisav-B)	Vitamins and mineral salts, yeast protein, yeast DNA, deoxycholate, phosphorothioate linked oligodeoxynucleotide, phosphate buffered saline, sodium phosphate, dibasic dodecahydrate, monobasic dehydrate, polysorbate 80
Hep A/Hep B (Twinrix)	MRC-5 human diploid cells, formalin, aluminum phosphate, aluminum hydroxide, amino acids, sodium chloride, phosphate buffer, polysorbate 20, neomycin sulfate, yeast protein
Human Papillomavirus (HPV) (Gardasil 9)	Vitamins, amino acids, mineral salts, carbohydrates, amorphous aluminum hydroxyphosphate sulfate, sodium chloride, L-histidine, polysorbate 80, sodium borate, yeast protein
Influenza (Afluria) Trivalent & Quadrivalent	Sodium chloride, monobasic sodium phosphate, dibasic sodium phosphate, monobasic potassium phosphate, potassium chloride, calcium chloride, sodium taurodeoxycholate, ovalbumin, sucrose, neomycin sulfate, polymyxin B, beta-propiolactone, thimerosal (multidose vials)
Influenza (Fluad)	Squalene, polysorbate 80, sorbitan trioleate, sodium citrate dehydrate, citric acid monohydrate, neomycin, kanamycin, barium, egg proteins, cetyltrimethylammonium bromide (CTAB), formaldehyde
Influenza (Fluarix) Trivalent & Quadrivalent	Octoxynol-10 (TRITON X-100), α-tocopheryl hydrogen succinate, polysorbate 80 (Tween 80), hydrocortisone, gentamicin sulfate, ovalbumin, formaldehyde, sodium deoxycholate, sodium phosphate-buffered isotonic sodium chloride
Influenza (Flublok) Trivalent & Quadrivalent	Sodium chloride, monobasic sodium phosphate, dibasic sodium phosphate, polysorbate 20 (Tween 20), baculovirus and Spodoptera frugiperda cell proteins, baculovirus and cellular DNA, Triton X-100, lipids, vitamins, amino acids, mineral salts
Influenza (Flucelvax) Trivalent & Quadrivalent	Madin Darby Canine Kidney (MDCK) cell protein, protein other than HA, MDCK cell DNA, polysorbate 80, cetyltrimethylammonium bromide, and β-propiolactone

Influenza (Flulaval) Trivalent & Quadrivalent	Ovalbumin, formaldehyde, sodium deoxycholate, α-tocopheryl hydrogen succinate, polysorbate 80, thimerosal (multi-dose vials)
Influenza (Fluvirin)	Ovalbumin, polymyxin, neomycin, betapropiolactone. nonyl-phenol ethoxylate, thimerosal
Influenza (Fluzone) Quadrivalent	Formaldehyde, egg protein, octylphenol ethoxylate (Triton X-100), sodium phosphate-buffered isotonic sodium chloride solution, thimerosal (multi-close vials) sucrose
Influenza (Fluzone) High Dose	Egg protein, octylphenol ethoxylate (Triton X-100), sodium phosphate-buffered isotonic sodium chloride solution, formalde-hyde, sucrose
Influenza (Fluzone) Intradermal	Egg protein, octylpnenol ethoxylate (Trinton X-100), sodium phosphate-buffered isotonic sodium chloride solution, sucrose
Influenza (FluMist) Quadrivalent	Monosodium glutamate, hydrolyzed porcine gelatin, arginine, sucrose, dibasic potassium phosphate, monobasic potassium phos-phate, ovalbumin, gentamicin sulfate, ethylenediaminetetraacetic acid (EDTA)
Japanese Encephalitis (Ixiaro)	Aluminum hydroxide, protamine sulfate, formaldehyde, bovine serum albumin, host cell DNA, sodium metabisulphite, host cell protein
Meningococcal (McnAC WY-Menactra)	Watson Scherp media containing casamino acid, modified cul-ture medium containing hydrolyzed casein, ammonium sulfate, sodium phosphate, formaldehyde, sodium chloride
Meningococcal (MenACWY-Menveo)	Formaldehyde, amino acids, yeast extract, Franz complete medium, CY medium
Meningococcal (MenB-Bexsero)	Aluminum hydroxide, E. coli, histidine, sucrose, deoxycholate, kanamycin
Meningococcal (MenB-Trumenba)	Defined fermentation growth media, polysorbate 80, histidine buffered saline
MMR (MMR-II)	Chick embryo cell culture, WI-38 human diploid lung fibro-blasts, vitamins, amino acids, fetal bovine serum, sucrose, gluta-mate, recombinant human albumin, neomycin, sorbitol, hydro-lyzed gelatin, sodium phosphate, sodium chloride
MMRV (ProQuad) (Frozen)	Chick embryo cell culture, WI-38 human diploid lung fibro-blasts, MRC-5 cells, sucrose, hydrolyzed gelatin, sodium chlo-ride, sorbitol, monosodium L-glutamate, sodium phosphate dibasic, human albumin, sodium bicarbonate, potassium phos-phate monobasic, potassium chloride; potassium phosphate diba-sic, neomycin, bovine calf serum

MMRV (ProQuad) (Refrigerator Stable)	Chick embryo cell culture, WI-38 human diploid lung fibroblasts, MRC-5 cells, sucrose, hydrolyzed gelatin, urea, sodium chloride, sorbitol, monosodium L-glutamate, sodium phosphate, recombinant human albumin, sodium bicarbonate, potassium phosphate, potassium chloride, neomycin, bovine serum albumin
Pneumococcal (PCV13-Prevnar 13)	Soy peptone broth, casamino acids and yeast extract-based medium, CRM197 carrier protein, polysorbate 80, succinate buffer, aluminum phosphate
Pneumococcal (PPSV-23-Pneumovax)	Phenol
Polio (IPV-Ipol)	Eagle MEM modified medium, calf bovine serum, M-199 without calf bovine serum, vero cells (a continuous line of monkey kidney cells), phenoxyethanol, formaldehyde, neomycin, streptomycin, polymyxin B
Rabies (Imovax)	Human albumin, neomycin sulfate, phenol red indicator, MRC-5 human diploid cells, beta-propriolactone
Rabies (RabAvert)	Chicken fibroblasts, P-propiolactone, polygeline (processed bovine gelatin), human serum albumin, bovine scram, potassium glutamate, sodium EDTA, ovalbumin, neomycin, chlortetracycline, amphotericin B
Rotavirus (RotaTeq)	Sucrose, sodium citrate, sodium phosphate monobasic monohydrate, sodium hydroxide, polysorbate 80, cell culture media, fetal bovine serum, vero cells [DNA from porcine circoviruses (PCV) 1 and 2 has been detected in RotaTeq. PCV-1 and PCV-2 are not known to cause disease in humans.]
Rotavirus (Rotarix)	Ammo acids, dextran, Dulbecco's Modified Eagle Medium (sodium chloride, potassium chloride, magnesium sulfate, ferric (XII) nitrate, sodium phosphate, sodium pyruvate, D-glucose, concentrated vitamin solution, L-cystine, L-tyrosine, amino acids solution, L-250 glutamine, calcium chloride, sodium hydrogenocarbonate, and phenol red), sorbitol, sucrose, calcium carbonate, sterile water, xanthan [Porcine circovirus type 1 (PCV-1) is present in Rotarix. PCV-l is not known to cause disease in humans.]
Smallpox (Vaccinia) (ACAM2000)	African Green Monkey kidney (Vero) cells, HEPES, human serum albumin, sodium chloride, neomycin, polymyxin B, Glycerin, phenol
Td (Tenivac)	aluminum phosphate, formaldehyde, modified Mueller-Miller casamino acid medium without beef heart infusion, ammonium sulfate

Td (Mass Biologics)	Aluminum phosphate, formaldehyde, thimerosal, modified Mueller's media which contains bovine extracts, ammonium sulfate
Tdap (Adacel)	Aluminum phosphate, formaldehyde, 2-phenoxyethanol, Stainer-Scholte medium, casamino acids, dimethyl-beta-cyclo-dextrin, glutaraldehyde, modified Mueller-Miller casamino acid medium without beef heart infusion, ammonium sulfate, modified Mueller's growth medium
Tdap (Boostrix)	Modified Latham medium derived from bovine casein, Fenton medium containing a bovine extract, formaldehyde, modified Stainer-Scholte liquid medium, glutaraldehyde, aluminum hydroxide, sodium chloride, polysorbate 80
Typhoid (Typhim Vi)	Hexadecyltrimethylammonium bromide, formaldehyde, phenol, polydimethylsiloxane, disodium phosphate, monosodium phosphate, semi-synthetic medium
Typhoid (Vivotif Ty2la)	Yeast extract, casein, dextrose, galactose, sucrose, ascorbic acid, amino acids, lactose, magnesium stearate, gelatin
Varicella (Varivax) Frozen	Human embryonic lung cell cultures, guinea pig cell cultures, human diploid cell cultures (WI-38), human diploid cell cultures (MRC-5), sucrose, hydrolyzed gelatin, sodium chloride, monosodium L-glutamate, sodium phosphate dibasic, potassium phosphate monobasic, potassium chloride, EDTA (Ethylcnediaminetetraacetic acid), neomycin, fetal bovine serum
Varicella (Varivax) Refrigerator Stable	Human embryonic lung cell cultures, guinea pig cell cultures, human diploid cell cultures (WI-38), human diploid cell cultures (MRC-5), sucrose, hydrolyzed gelatin, urea, sodium chloride, monosodium L-glutamate, sodium phosphate dibasic, potassium phosphate monobasic, potassium chloride, neomycin, bovine calf serum
Yellow Fever (YF-Vax)	sorbitol, gelatin, sodium chloride, egg protein
Zoster (Shingles) (Zostavax) Frozen	Sucrose, hydrolyzed porcine gelatin, sodium chloride, monosodium L-glutamate, sodium phosphate dibasic, potassium phosphate monobasic, potassium chloride; MRC-5 cells, neomycin, bovine calf serum
Zoster (Shingles) (Zostavax) Refrigerator Stable	Sucrose, hydrolyzed porcine gelatin, urea, sodium chloride, monosodium L-glutamate, sodium phosphate dibasic, potassium phosphate monobasic, potassium chloride, MRC-5 cells, neomycin, bovine calf serum

Zoster (Shingles) (Shingrix)	Sucrose, sodium chloride, dioleoyl phosphatidylcholine (DOPC), potassium dihydrogen phosphate, cholesterol, sodium dihydrogen phosphate dihydrate, disodium phosphate anhydrous, dipotassium phosphate, polysorbate 80, Chinese Hamster Ovary (CHO) cell proteins, DNA

A table listing vaccine excipients and media by excipient can be found in: Grabenstein JD. ImmunoFacts: Vaccines and Immunologic Drugs—2013 (38th revision). St Louis, MO: Wolters Kluwer Health, 2012. March 2018

DEFINITIONS OF VACCINE INGREDIENTS

In Opposition to the Ways of the Bible

- Human diploid fibroblast cell cultures (stain WI-38): lung tissue of an aborted three-month female fetus
- Fetal Bovine Serum: an amber-colored, protein-rich liquid that separates out when blood coagulates, from a baby cow
- Human serum albumin: the primary protein present in human blood plasma
- Human diploid cell cultures: human embryonic lung cell cultures. There are two human diploid cell lines which were originally prepared from tissues of aborted fetuses and are used for the preparation of vaccines based on live attenuated virus. The first one is the WI-38, with human diploid lung fibroblasts, coming from a female fetus that was aborted. The second human cell line is MRC-5, with human lung fibroblasts coming from an aborted fourteen-week male fetus.
- Formaldehyde: a colorless poisonous gas; made by the oxidation of methanol. Pneumonia and bronchitis are found in all animals after the injection of formalin, a carcinogenic.
- Formalin: a 37 percent aqueous (water) solution of formaldehyde, a pungent gas
- Aluminum phosphate: may contribute to the onset of Alzheimer's disease. Exposure to this chemical is quite harmful and would require serious medical attention if ingestion or contact occurs.

- Ammonium sulfate: It can cause severe irritation and inflammation to the respiratory tract. Eating or drinking ammonium sulfate will cause irritation in the gastrointestinal tract like nausea, vomiting, and diarrhea.
- Bovine extract: pituitary gland from cattle. Risk of exposure to infectious agents, including those that cause "mad cow disease." Prions—pertinacious infectious particles—are misshapen or misfolded protiens which, when introduced into your tissues, can induce your normal proteins to assume the misfolded state. Although they are not viruses, prions behave like viruses in that they can serve as templates to trigger a chain reaction of prion formation in your tissues, most notable in your brain.
- Vero cells: derived from the kidney of an African green monkey
- DNA from porcine circoviruses
- PCV-X and PCV-2: Porcine cirovirus is a group of single-stranded DNA viruses, that is nonenveloped with an unsegmented circular genome
- Fetal bovine serum: calf serum. Fetal bovine serum comes from the blood drawn from a bovine fetus via a closed system of collection at the slaughterhouse.
- MRC-5 cells: (Medical Research Council cell strain 5) is a diploid human cell culture line composed of fibroblasts derived from lung tissue of a fourteen-week-old aborted Caucasian male fetus.
- Normal human diploid cells: WI-38 is a diploid human cell strain composed of fibroblasts derived from lung tissue of a three-month aborted female fetus.
- Bovine serum albumin: BSA or Fraction V is a serum albumin protein derived from cows.
- Bovine extract is derived from the pituitary gland, a small endocrine gland that produces and secretes various hormones that are vital to the regulation of various bodily functions.
- Aluminum hydroxide
- Amorphous aluminum hydroxyphosphate sulfate: Aluminium adjuvants remain the most widely used and effective adjuvants in vaccination and immunotherapy. Herein, the particle size

distribution (PSD) of aluminium oxyhydroxide and aluminium hydroxyphosphate adjuvants was elucidated in attempt to correlate these properties with the biological responses observed post vaccination. Heightened solubility and potentially the generation of A13+ in the lysosomal environment were positively correlated with an increase in cell mortality in vitro, potentially generating a greater inflammatory response at the site of simulated injection. The cellular uptake of aluminium based adjuvants (ABAs) used in clinically approved vaccinations are compared to a commonly used experimental ABA, in an in vitro THP-1 cell model. Using lumogallion as a direct-fluorescent molecular probe for aluminium, complemented with transmission electron microscopy of internalized particulates, driven by the physicochemical variations of the ABAs investigated. We demonstrate that not all aluminium adjuvants are equal neither in terms of their physical properties nor their biological reactivity and potential toxicities both at the injection site and beyond. High loading of aluminium oxyhydroxide in the cytoplasm of THP-1 cells without immediate cytotoxicity might predispose this form of aluminium adjuvant to its subsequent transport throughout the body including access to the brain.

- Aluminium based adjuvants (ABA) are included in human vaccinations to boost or potentiate the immune response, to the injected antigen. Whilst a consensus upon the immunomodulatory mechanism of action of ABA has yet to be reached, it has become increasingly recognized that activation of the innate immune response is crucial for increased antibody titres. The continued and widespread use of ABA has followed the emergence of recombinant expressed protein antigens of high purity as a safer alternative to inactivated or attenuated pathogens. Owing to the homogeneity and generally weak immunogenic of recombinant antigens, the inclusion of adjuvants is often necessary for the induction of robust immune responses and effective immunization. Furthermore, the use of adjuvants in human vaccinations has been linked to adverse effects often classified under Autoimmune (or auto inflammatory) syndrome induced by adjuvants (ASIA). Combined with the relatively low cost of hydrated colloidal aluminium salts and their ease of inclusion as effective adjuvants within clinically approved vaccine formulations, the continued use of ABA in human vaccinations is likely to continue.

- Of the most commonly used ABA in clinically approved vaccine formulations are the commercially available aluminium oxyhydroxide based, Alhydrogel and aluminium hydroxyphosphate based, Adju-Phos, adjuvants. More recently a sulphated derivative of the latter in the form of aluminium hydroxyphosphate sulpate has been used as a single component of an adjuvant system against human papilloma virus (HPV). Typically, the adsorptive capacity of an ABA to its antigen, dictate its choice in studies of adjuvant city. In this respect, the choice of adjuvants is selected according to its zeta potential or surface charge of which Alhydrogel is positively charged at neutral pH and suitable for adsorption to negatively charged antigens, conversely to negatively charged particulates of Adju-Phos. Ovalbumin is frequently used as a model protein antigen in experimental vaccine formulations and owing to its number of side-chain carboxyl groups, possesses a net negative charge. As such, Alhydrogel continues to predominate as the clinically relevant adjuvant of choice in the studies.
- (ncbl.nlm.nih.gov) National Center for Biotechnology Information
- Polysorbate 80
- Polysorbate 20 is fragrance component, a surfactant, an emulsifying agent, and a solubilizing agent. Polysorbate starts out as harmless sorbitol, but then it's treated with carcinogenic ethylene oxide. It's called Polysorbate 20 because it's treated with 20 "parts" of ethylene oxide.
- DNA: deoxyribonucleic acid, a self-replicating material which is present in nearly all living organisms as the main constituent of chromosomes. It is the carrier of genetic information.
- Ovalbumin: is the main protein found in egg white, making up approximately 55% of the total protein.
- Thiomersal:

- Thimerosal is an organo mercury compound. This compound is a well-established antiseptic and antifungal agent. Thimerosal is very toxic by inhalation, ingestion, and in contact with skin, with a danger of cumulative effects. It is also very toxic to aquatic organisms and may cause long-term adverse effects in aquatic environments. In the body, it is metabolized or degraded to Ethylmercury and Thiosalicylate.
- WI-38 human diploid lung fibroblasts: a diploid human cell strain composed of fibroblasts derived from lung tissue of an aborted three-month female fetus.
- Recombinant Human Albumin is a highly purified animal-, virus-, and prion-free product developed as an alternative to human serum albumin (HAS), to which it is structurally equivalent.
- Human Serum Albumin
- Human Albumin is the serum albumin found in human blood. It is the most abundant protein in human blood plasma; it constitutes about half of serum protein. It is produced in the liver. It is soluble in water and monomeric.
- Chinese Hamster Ovary (CHO) cell proteins: an epithelial cell line derived from the ovary of the Chinese hamster, often used in biological and medical research and commercially in the production of therapeutic proteins.
- Canine Kidney cell DNA (MDCK): derived from the kidney tissue of an adult female cocker spaniel.
- E. coli: Escherichia coli, bacteria normally living in the intestines of healthy people and animals. Most varieties of E. coli are harmless or cause relatively brief diarrhea. But a few particularly nasty strains, can cause severe abdominal cramps, bloody diarrhea and vomiting.
- Chick embryo cell culture
- Chicken Fibroblasts: The technique, which requires cutting the skin off the embryo, or using skin of intact chicken embryos.
- Guinea Pig cell cultures: an alternative cell culture system for the isolation and propagation of certain types of group A coxsackieviruses.

- Host cell DNA: A cell that harbors foreign molecules, viruses, or microorganisms. For example, a cell being host to a virus. A cell that has been introduced with DNA or RNA, such as a bacterial cell acting as a host cell for the DNA isolated from a bacteriophage.

BIBLICAL SCRIPTURES

- "You shall not murder" (Exodus 20:13).
- "You shall not murder" (Deuteronomy 5:17).
- "Adam made love to his wife Eve, and she became pregnant and gave birth to Cain. She said, 'With the help of the Lord I have brought forth a man'" (Genesis 4:1).
- "Before I formed you in the womb I knew you, before you were born I set you apart; I appointed you as a prophet to the nations" (Jeremiah 1:5).
- "For you created my inmost being; you knit me together in my mother's womb. I praise you because I am fearfully and wonderfully made; your works are wonderful, I know that full well. My frame was not hidden from you when I was made in the secret place, when I was woven together in the depths of the earth. Your eyes saw my unformed body; all the days ordained for me were written in your book before one of them came to be" (Psalm 139:13–16).
- "From birth I was cast on you; from my mother's womb you have been my God. Do not be far from me, for trouble is near and there is no one to help" (Psalm 22:10–11).
- "God blessed them and said to them, 'Be fruitful and increase in number; fill the earth and subdue it. Rule over the fish in the sea and the birds in the sky and over every living creature that moves on the ground'" (Genesis 1:28).
- "Children are a heritage from the Lord, offspring a reward from him" (Psalm 127:3).
- "He raises the poor from the dust and lifts the needy from the ash heap; he seats them with princes, with the princes of his people. He settles the childless woman in her home as a happy mother of children. Praise the Lord" (Psalm 113:7–9).

- "At that time the disciples came to Jesus and asked, 'Who, then, is the greatest in the kingdom of heaven?' He called a little child to him, and placed the child among them, and he said: 'Truly I tell you, unless you change and become like little children, you will never enter the kingdom of heaven. Therefore, whoever takes the lowly position of his child is the greatest in the kingdom of heaven, and whoever welcomes one such child in my name welcomes me. If anyone causes one of these little ones—those who believe in me—to stumble, it would be better for them to have a large millstone hung around their neck and to be drowned in the depths of the sea. Woe to the world because of the things that cause people to stumble, it would be better for them to have a large millstone hung around their neck and to be drowned in the depths of the sea. Woe to the world because of the things that cause people to stumble! Such things must come, but woe to the person through whom they come! If your hand or your foot causes you to stumble, cut it off and throw it away. It is better for you to enter life maimed or crippled than to have two hands or two feet and be thrown into eternal fire. And if your eye causes you to stumble, gouge it out and throw it away. It is better for you to enter life with one eye than to have two eyes and be thrown into the fire of hell. See that you do not despise one of these little ones. For I tell you that their angels in heaven always see the face of my Father in heaven. What do you think? If a man owns a hundred sheep, and one of them wanders away, will he not leave the ninety-nine on the hills and go to look for the one that wandered off? And if he finds it, truly I tell you, he is happier about that one sheep than about the ninety-nine that did not wander off. In the same way your Father in heaven is not willing that any of these little ones should perish'" (Matthew 18:1–14).
- "Then people brought little children to Jesus for him to place his hands on them and pray for them. But the disciples rebuked them. Jesus said, 'Let the little children come to me, and do not hinder them, for the kingdom of heaven belongs to such as these' When he had placed his hands on them, he went on from there" (Matthew 19:13–15).

- "So God created mankind in his own image, in the image of God he created them; male and female he created them" (Genesis 1:27).
- "But they mingled with the nations and adopted their customs. They sacrificed their sons and their daughters to false gods. They shed innocent blood, the blood of their sons and daughters, whom they sacrificed to the idols of Canann, and the land was desecrated by their blood" (Psalm 106:35, 37–38).
- "This is what the Lord says: 'For three sins of Ammon, even for four, I will not relent. Because he ripped open the pregnant women of Gilead in order to extend his borders'" (Amos 1:13).
- "They sacrificed their sons and daughters in the fire. They practiced divination and sought omens and sold themselves to do evil in the eyes of the Lord, arousing his anger. So the Lord was very angry with Israel and removed them from his presence. Only the tribe of Judah was left" (2 Kings 17:17–18).
- "Do you not know that your bodies are temples of the Holy Spirit, who is in you, whom you have received from God? You are not your own; you were bought at a price. Therefore honor God with your bodies" (1 Corinthians 6:19–20).
- "But you must not eat meat that has its lifeblood still in it" (Genesis 9:4).
- "I will set my face against any Israelite or any foreigner residing among them who eats blood, and I will cut them off from the people. For the life of a creature is in the blood, and I have given it to you to make atonement for yourselves on the altar; it is the blood that makes atonement for one's life. Because the life of every creature is its blood. That is why I have said to the Israelites, 'You must not eat the blood of any creature, because the life of every creature is its blood; anyone who eats it must be cut off'" (Leviticus 17:10–11, 14).
- "But be sure you do not eat the blood, because the blood is the life, and you must not eat the life with the meat" (Deuteronomy 12:23).
- "Instead we should write to them, telling them to abstain from food polluted by idols, from sexual immorality, from the meat

of strangled animals and from blood. You are to abstain from food sacrificed to idols, from blood, from the meat of strangled animals and from sexual immorality. You will do well to avoid these things. Farewell" (Acts 15:20, 29).

- "And after they have been destroyed before you, be careful not to be ensnared by inquiring about their gods, saying, "How do these nations serve their gods? We will do the same." You must not worship the LORD your God in their way, because in worshiping their gods, they do all kinds of detestable things the LORD hates. They even burn their sons and daughters in the fire as sacrifices to their gods. See that you do all I command you; do not add to it or take away from it" (Deuteronomy 12:30–32).
- "Let no one be found among you who sacrifices their son or daughter in the fire, who practices divination or sorcery, interprets omens, engages in witchcraft" (Deuteronomy 18:10).
- "Ahaz was twenty years old when he became king, and he reigned in Jerusalem sixteen years. Unlike David his father, he did not do what was right in the eyes of the LORD his God. He followed the ways of the kings of Israel and even sacrificed his son in the fire, engaging in the detestable practices of the nations the LORD had driven out before the Israelites" (2 Kings 16:2–3).
- "They shed innocent blood, the blood of their sons and daughters, whom they sacrificed to the idols of Canaan, and the land was desecrated by their blood" (Psalm 106:38).
- "Do not give any of your children to be sacrificed to Molek, for you must not profane the name of your God. I am the LORD" (Leviticus 18:21).
- "The LORD said to Moses, 'Say to the Israelites: Any Israelite or any foreigner residing in Israel who sacrifices any of his children to Molek is to be put to death. The members of the community are to stone him. I myself will set my face against him and will cut him off from his people; for by sacrificing his children to Molek, he has defiled my sanctuary and profaned my holy name. If the members of the community close their eyes when that man sacrifices one of his children to Molek and if they fail to put him to death, I myself will set my face against him and his

family and will cut them off from their people together with all who follow him in prostituting themselves to Molek'" (Leviticus 20:2–5).

- "Trust in the LORD with all your heart and lean not on your own understanding; in all your ways submit to him, and he will make your paths straight" (Proverbs 3:5–6).

- "For the entire law is fulfilled in keeping this one command: 'Love your neighbor as yourself.' If you bite and devour each other, watch out or you will be destroyed by each other. So I say, walk by the Spirit, and you will not gratify the desires of the flesh. For the flesh desires what is contrary to the Spirit, and the Spirit what is contrary to the flesh. They are in conflict with each other, so that you are not to do whatever you want. But if you are led by the Spirit, you are not under the law. The acts of the flesh are obvious: sexual immorality, impurity and debauchery; idolatry and witchcraft; hatred, discord, jealousy, fits of rage, selfish ambitions, dissensions, factions and envy; drunkenness, orgies, and the like. I warn you, as I did before, that those who live like this will not inherit the kingdom of God" (Galatians 5:14–21).

- "Nor did they repent of their murders, their magic arts, their sexual immorality or their thefts" (Revelations 9:21).

- "The light of a lamp will never shine in you again. The voice of bridegroom and bride will never be heard in you again. Your merchants were the world's important people. By your magic spell all the nations were led astray" (Revelations 18:23).

- "But the cowardly, the unbelieving, the vile, the murderers, the sexually immoral, those who practice magic arts, the idolaters and all liars—they will be consigned to the fiery lake of burning sulfur. This is the second death" (Revelations 21:8).

- "Outside are the dogs, those who practice magic arts, the sexually immoral, the murderers, the idolaters and everyone who loves and practices falsehood. 'I, Jesus, have sent my angel to give you this testimony for the churches. I am the Root and the Offspring of David, and the bright Morning Star'" (Revelations 22:15–16).

HUMAN AND ANIMAL VACCINE CONTAMINATIONS

Abstract

Vaccination is one of the most important public health accomplishments. However, since vaccine preparation involves the use of materials of biological origin, vaccines are subject to contamination by micro-organisms. In fact, vaccine contamination has occurred; a historical example of vaccine contamination, for example, can be found in the early days of development of the smallpox vaccine. The introduction of new techniques of vaccine virus production on cell cultures has led to safer vaccines, but has not completely removed the risk of virus contamination. There are several examples of vaccine contamination, for example, contamination of human vaccines against poliomyelitis by SV40 virus from the use of monkey primary renal cells. Several veterinary vaccines have been contaminated by pestiviruses from foetal calf serum. These incidents have lead industry to change certain practices and regulatory authorities to develop more stringent and detailed requirements. But the increasing number of target species for vaccines, the diversity of the origin of biological materials and the extremely high number of known and unknown viruses and their constant evolution represent a challenge to vaccine producers and regulatory authorities.

RISKS OF LIVE VIRUS AND VECTORED VACCINES

What I am about to share with you is factual referenced reports from the National Vaccine Information Center. The emerging risks of live virus and virus-vectored vaccines (any agent, person, or animal or microorganism that carries and transmits a disease) are real. I will be sharing about vaccine strain virus infection, shedding, and transmission.

For more in-depth articles, please visit www.NVIC.org. Your health. Your family. Your choice.

Can people receiving live virus vaccines transmit vaccine strain virus to others? Could my unvaccinated or immune compromised child get sick from coming in contact with a recently vaccinated person? *Yes.* When you experience a viral infection, live virus is shed in the body fluids of those who are infected for different amounts of time and can be transmitted to others.[1, 2, 3] Vaccine strain live virus is also shed for different amounts of time in the body fluids of vaccinated people and can be transmitted to others.[4, 5, 6] Even though public health officials maintain that live attenuated, weakened, virus vaccines rarely cause complications in the person vaccinated and that vaccine strain viral shedding rarely causes disease in close contacts of the recently vaccinated, it is important to be aware that vaccine strain live virus infection can sometimes cause serious complications in vaccinated persons and vaccine strain live viruses can be shed and transmitted to others with serious or even fatal consequences.

How will shedding with GMO virus-vectored vaccines affect us? Humans and animals receiving certain live virus-vectored vaccines will be shedding and transmitting genetically modified vaccine strains that may pose unpredictable risks to the vaccinated, close contacts and environment. For example, vaccine developers creating an experimental AIDS vaccine by genetically engineering the live-attenuated measles virus to express a fusion protein containing HIV-1 antigens face challenges in trying to limit shedding and transmission of infectious virus by the recently vaccinated.[7] These very real risks should be thoroughly quantified before licensure and widespread use of GMO vaccine[8] because the ability of vaccine strain viruses to recombine with wild-type viruses and produce new hybrid viruses with potentially serious side effects that are shed and transmitted in human and animal populations cannot be underestimated.[9, 10]

There is an urgent need to apply precautionary principle. There are important unanswered questions about the effect that widespread use of live virus vaccines have had in the past and the genetically modified virus-vectored vaccines will have in the future on epigenetic, the integrity of the micro biome, human health, and environmental ecosystems.[11, 12]

As several Norwegian scientists warned in 2012, "Genetically engineered or modified viruses (GMVs) are being increasingly used as live vaccine vectors and their applications may have environmental implications that must be taken into account in risk assessment and management processes. In all cases there may be circumstances that enable GMVs to jump species barriers directly, or following recombination with naturally occurring viruses. All the different applications may, to varying extents, represent release of unintended escape of GMVs into the highly varying ecosystems."[13] In light of long standing, significant gaps in scientific knowledge about infectious microbes, the micro biome, epigenetic and the nature of human health, the long-term safety and effectiveness of using live attenuated virus vaccines and genetically modifies virus-vectored vaccines has not yet been established.[14, 15, 16]

Let's talk about viral infections, shedding, and transmission. Humans experience and recover from many different types of viral infections from infancy and throughout life without suffering chronic health problems. Common respiratory and gastrointestinal symptoms of viral infections include fever, sore throat, runny nose, coughing, headache, diarrhea, vomiting, and other symptoms that usually resolve without causing harm. However, depending upon the virus and the health of a person, serious complications of viral infections can include dehydration, secondary bacterial infections, brain inflammation, shock, and death. People at higher risk of viral infection complications include infants, the elderly, and those with compromised immune system, malnutrition, and living in unsanitary conditions, lack of sleep and high levels of stress, and history of chronic disease. People shed for different lengths of time. When someone has a viral infection that causes illness, that person can shed and transmit virus for different lengths of time depending upon the virus and the health or other individual characteristics of the infected person.[17] Viruses are shed and transmitted through coughing and sneezing, exchange of saliva (kissing or sharing drinking cups), skin-to-skin contact (for example, touching chickenpox lesions), breast milk and exposure to blood, urine or feces (changing a baby's diapers), semen, or other body fluids. Smallpox, polio, measles, mumps, rubella, influenza, rotavirus, chicken pox, and shingles are viral infectious diseases for which live virus vaccines have been widely used by human populations for the past century.

There are different types of vaccines, including vaccines containing inactivated (killed) microbes and those containing live attenuated viruses.[18, 19] Live attenuated viral vaccines are created in a number of ways; but one of the most common methods involves passing a virus through a living cell culture or host (such as chicken embryo, monkey or dog kidney cells, human fetal lung cells) over and over until there is a reduced risk the weakened virus will make a person seriously ill but is still capable of stimulating a strong enough inflammatory response in the body to produce vaccine acquired antibodies.[20] Sometimes, the weakened vaccine strain live virus can mutate and regain virulence, extreme harmfulness with the capacity of a microorganism to cause disease. This includes neurovirulence, which significantly raises risks of serious complications from vaccine strain virus infection.[21, 22] Healthy persons can suffer complications from vaccine strain viral infection,[23] but children and adults with immunodeficiency are more likely to develop complications after they receive live virus vaccines or come in close contact with a person who is shedding vaccine strain live virus.[24, 25] The live virus vaccines currently recommended by public health officials in the US include measles-mumps-rubella (MMR), varicella (chickenpox), influenza (nasal spray), rotavirus, and herpes zoster (shingles) vaccines. Other live, attenuated vaccines licensed in the US but which are not currently recommended for routine use in the US include adenovirus,[26] yellow fever, smallpox, typhoid, and oral polio vaccines.[27]

Vaccine strain live virus can infect others. Just like people with viral infections can shed and transmit wild-type virus,[28] people given live virus vaccines can shed and transmit vaccine strain live attenuated virus.[29] Like wild-type, vaccine strain live virus can be shed in body fluids, such as saliva,[30, 31] nasal and throat secretions,[32] breast milk,[33, 34] urine and blood,[35, 36] stool,[37] and skin lesions.[38] Shedding after vaccination with live virus vaccines may continue for days, weeks, or months, depending upon the vaccine and the health or other individual host factors of the vaccinated person.

Many people with viral infections have no clinical symptoms. One of the big problems with diagnosing illness is that both vaccinated and unvaccinated people can experience and recover from a viral infection, including shedding infectious virus[39, 40] but show only mild or no clinical symptoms.[41, 42, 43, 44] (Bacterial infections like B. pertussis whooping cough can also be transmitted by vaccinated or unvaccinated persons showing no symptoms.[45, 46]) Outside of the medical community, there is little public awareness about the fact that you can be infected with shed and transmit wild-type virus or vaccine strain live virus without having any symptoms at all.

For more in-depth, scientific, research reports, please reference NVIC referenced report. Topic to search is *The Emerging Risks of Live Virus and Virus Vectored Vaccines.*

SAMPLE REQUEST FOR RELIGIOUS EXEMPTION TO IMMUNIZATION FORM

Parent/Guardian Statement

Name of student
Identification number
Name of parent(s)/guardian(s)
School district and building name

This form is for your use in applying for a religious exemption to Public Health Law immunization requirements for your child. Its purpose is to establish the religious basis for your request since the state permits exemptions on the basis of a sincere religious belief philosophical, political, scientific, or sociological objections to immunization do not justify an exemption under Department of Health regulation 10 NYCRR, Section 66–1.3 (d), which requires the submission of:

A written and signed statement from the parent, parents, or guardian of such child, stating that the parent, parents or guardian objects to their child's immunization due to sincere and genuine religious beliefs which prohibit the immunization of their child in which case the principal or person in charge may require supporting documents.

In the area provided below, please write your statement. The statement must address all of the following elements:

- Explain in your own words why you are requesting this religious exemption.
- Describe the religious principles that guide your objection to immunization.
- Indicate whether you are opposed to all immunizations and if not the religious basis that prohibits particular immunizations.

You may attach to this form additional written pages or other supporting materials if you so choose. Examples of such materials are listed on page 3.

Please sign in the space provided below.

I hereby affirm the truthfulness of the forgoing statement and have received and reviewed the informational immunization materials provided to me by my child's school.

Signature of parent/guardian
Date

You will be notified in writing of the outcome of this request. Please note that if your request for an exemption is denied, you may appeal the denial to the Commissioner of Education within thirty (30) days of the decision, pursuant to Education Law, Section 310.
March 2016

SECTION BELOW FOR SCHOOL DISTRICT USE ONLY

To the building principal:

If, after review of the parental statement, questions remain about the existence of a sincerely held religious belief, Department of Health regulation [10 NYCRR, Section 66-1.3(d)] permits the principal to request supporting documents. Some examples include:

- A letter from an authorized representative of the church, temple, religious institution, etc. attended by the parent/guardian, literature from the church, temple, religious institution, etc. explaining doctrine/beliefs that prohibit immunization (Note: Parents/guardians need not necessarily be a member of an organized religion or religious institution to obtain a religious exemption);
- Other writings or sources upon which the parent/guardian relied in formulating religious beliefs that prohibit immunization;
- A copy of any parental/guardian statements to health care providers or school district officials in a district of prior residence explaining the religious basis for refusing immunization;
- Any documents or other information the parent/guardian may be willing to provide that reflect a sincerely held religious objection to immunization (for example: disclosure of whether parent/guardian or other children have been

immunized, parent/guardian's current position on allowing himself or herself or his or her children to receive or refuse other kinds of medical treatment).

Reviewer Name (building principal)
Indicate result of request review:

Approved
Date of approval
Denied
Date of denial
State specifically reason(s) for denial:
You may attach additional sheets if necessary.
Reviewer signature (building principal)

Parent/guardian mint be notified in writing of the approval or denial of the request. If the request is denied, the notification letter must Include the specific reason(s) for denial.

If a religious exemption request is denied, the parent/guardian may appeal the denial to the Commissioner of Education within thirty (30) days of decision, pursuant to Education Law, Section 310.

NOTES

[1] Baron S, Fons M, Albrecht T. Viral Pathogenesis. In: Medical Microbiology, 4th Edition. University of Texas Medical Branch at Galveston 1996.

[2] Schwartz RA. Enteroviruses. Medscape Sept. 11, 2014.

[3] NVIC.Org. Ebola (Ebola Hemorrhagic Fever).

[4] King JC, Treanor J, Fast PE et al. comparison of the Safety. Vaccine Virus Shedding and Immunogenicity of Influenza Virus Vaccine. Trivalent Types A and B. Live Cold-Adapted. Administered to Human Immunodeficiency Virus (HIV)-Infected and Non-HIV Infected Adults. J Infect Dis2000; 181(2): 725–728.

[5] Payne DC, Edwards KM, Bowen MD et al. Sibling Transmission of Vaccine-Derived Rotavirus (RotaTeq) Associated with Rotavirus Gastroenteritis. Pediatrics 2010; 125(2).

[6] Mckenna M. Polio vaccination may continue after wild virus fades. CIDRAP Oct. 16, 2008.

[7] Lorin C, Setal L, Mois Jet al. Toxicology, biodistribution and shedding profile of a recombinant measles vaccine vector expressing HIV-1 antigens, in cynomolgus macaques. Nurnyn-Schmiedebergis Arch Pharmacol 2012; 385.

[8] BioOutsource. Virus and Vector Shedding. 2014.

[9] Spaete RR. Recombinant Live Attenuated Viral Vaccines. In: New Vaccine Technologies 2001.

[10] Dahourou G, Guillot S, Le Gall O, Crainic R. Genetic recombination in wild-type poliovirus. J Gen Virol 2002; 83: 3103–3110.

[11] Sandvik T, Tryland M, Hansen H et al. Naturally Occurring Orthopoxviruses: Potential for Recombination with Vaccine Vectors. J Clin Microbiol 1998; 360. 2542–2547.

[12] Schaller B, Sandu N. Clinical medicine, public health and ecological health: a new basis for education and prevention? Arch Med Sci 2011; 7(4): 541–545.

[13] Myhr Al, Traavik T. Genetically Engineered Virus-Vectored Vaccines-Environmental Risk Assessment and Management Challenges. In: Genetic Engineering—Basics, New Applications and Responsibilities. In Tech 2012.

[14] Ibid.

[15] Souza APD, Haut L, Reyes-Sandoval A, Pinto AR. Recombinant viruses as vaccines against viral diseases. Braz J Med Biol Res 2005; 38: 509–522.

[16] Lauring AS, Jones JO, Andino R. Rationalizing the development of live attenuated virus vaccines. Nature Biotech 2010:28: 573–579.

[17] Barker J, Stevens D, Bloomfield SF. Spread and prevention of some common viral infections in community facilities and domestic homes. Journal of Applied Microbiology 2001; 91(1): 7–21.

[18] NIH. Types of Vaccines. NIAID April 3, 2012.

[19] Goldenthal KL, Midthun K, Zoon KC. Control of Viral Infections and Diseases. Medical Microbiology 4th edition (Chapter 51) 1996.

[20] Food and Drug Administration (FDA). Background on Viral Vaccine Development. Mar. 23, 2010.

[21] HistoryofVaccines.org. History of Vaccines: Different Types of Vaccines. A Project of the College of Physicians of Philadelphia. Updated Jan. 27, 2014.

[22] Valsamakis A, Auwaerter PG, Rima BK et al. Altered Virulence of Vaccine Strains of Measles Virus after Prolonged Replication in Human Tissue. J Virol 1999; 73(10): 8791–8797.

[23] Levin M, DeBiasi RL, Bistik V, Schmid DS. Herpes Zoster with Skin Lesions and Meningitis Caused by 2 Different Genotypes of the Oka Varicella-Zoster Virus Vaccine. J Infect Dis 2008; 198(1): 1444–1447.

[24] Bitnun A, Shannon P, Durward A et al. Measles Inclusion-Body Encephalitis Caused by the Vaccine Strain of Measles Virus. Clin Infect Dis 1999; 29: 855–861.

[25] Rubin LG, Levin MJ, Ljungman P et al. 2013 IPSA Clinical Practice Guidelines for Vaccination of the Immunocompromised Host. Recommendations for Vaccination of Household Members of Immunocompromised Patients. Clin Infect Dis Dec. 4, 2013.

[26] FDA. Adenovirus Type 4 and 7 Vaccine. Live. Oral Prescribing Information. Barr Labs 2011.

[27] Centers for Disease Control (CDC). U.S. Vaccines 2012. The Pink Book May 2012 (12th Edition).

[28] CDC. Ebola Transmission. Oct. 13, 2014.

[29] Vignuzzi M, Wendt E, Andino R. Engineering attenuated virus vaccines by controlling replication fidelity. Nature Medicine 2008:14(2): 154–161.

[30] Teichert E. Virus present UP to one month after Zostavax immunization. Fierce Vaccines Mar. 9, 2011.

[31] Gershon A A. The History and Mystery of VZV in Saliva. J Infect Dis 2011; 204(6): 815–816.

[32] Ali T, Scott N, Kallas W et al. Detection of Influenza Antigen with Rapid Antibody-Based Tests After Intranasal Influenza Vaccination (FluMist). Clin Infect Dis 2004; 38(5): 760–762.

[33] Alain S. Dommergues MA, Jacquard AC. State of the art: Could nursing mothers be vaccinated with attenuated live virus vaccine? Vaccine 2012; 30(33): 4921-4926.

34 FDA. MMRII (Measles. Mumps and rubella Virus Vaccine Live): Nursing Mothers. Merck & Co, Inc. December 2010.

35 Buimovici-Klein E, Cooper EZ. Immunosuppression and Isolation of Rubella Virus from Human Lymphocytes After Vaccination with Two Rubella Vaccines. Infection and Immunity 1979; 25(1): 352–356.

36 Eckerle I, Keller-Stanislawski B, Eis-Hubinger AM. Nonfebrile Seizures after Mumps. Measles. Rubella and Varicella-oster Virus Combination Vaccination with Detection of Measles Virus RNA in Serum. Throat and Urine. Clin Vaccine Immunol 2013; 29(7): 1094–1096.

37 Laassr M, Lottenback K, Beishe R et al. Effect of Different Vaccination Schedules on Excretion of Oral Poliovirus Vaccine Strains. J Infect Dis 2005; 192 (12): 2092–2098.

38 La Russa P, Steinberg S, Meurice F, Gershon A. Transmission of Vaccine Strain Varicella Zoster Virus from a Healthy Adult with Vaccine-Associated Rash to Susceptible Household Contacts. J Infect Dis 1997; 176:1072–1075.

39 Adalja AA. A Prospective Study of Influenza Shedding in the Community. Clinician's Biosecurity News Dec. 21, 2012.

40 Cohrs RJ, Mehta SK, Schmid DS et al. Asymptomatic Reactivation and Shed of Infectious Varicella Zoster Virus in Astronauts. J Med Virol 2008; 80(6): 1116-1122.

41 Rogers E. London study finds 77 percent of influenza infections are asymptomatic. Vaccine New Daily Mar. 20, 2014.

42 Carrat F, Vergu E, Ferguson NM. Time Lines of Infections and Disease in Human Influenza: A Review of Volunteer Challenge Studies. Am J Epidemiol 2008:167:775-785.

43 Feibelkorn AP, Barskey A, Hickman C, Bellini W. Mumps. In: Manual for surveillance of Vaccine Preventable Diseases. CDC April 1, 2014.

44 Pichichero ML, Losonsky GA. Asymptomatic infections due to wild-type rotavirus may prime for a heterotypic response to vaccination with rhesus rotavirus. Clin Infect Dis 1993; 16(1): 86–92.

45 Bakalar N. Study Finds Parents Can Pass Whooping Cough to Babies. New York Times April 3, 2007.

46 Warfel JM, Zimmerman LI, Merkel TJ. Acellular pertussis vaccines protect against disease but fail to prevent infection and transmission in a nonhuman primate model. Proc Natl Acad Sci 2014; 111(2): 787–792.

47 http://www.cdc.aov/vaccines/pubs/pinkbook/downloads/appendices/B/excipient-table-2.PDF

48 http://www.fda.aov/BiologicsBloodVaccines/Vaccines/ApprovedProducts/ucm093833.htm

49 https://www.ncbl.nlm.nih.aov/pubmed/20456974

50 https://www.livingwhole.ora/resources/

51 The Holy Bible, NIV

ABOUT THE AUTHOR

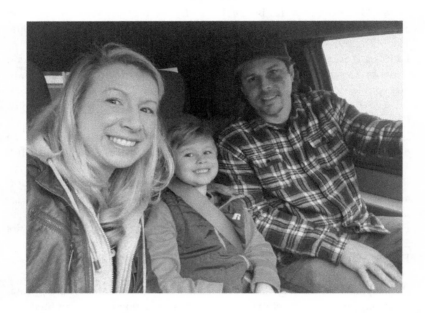

"But those who wait for the Lord shall change and renew their strength and power; they shall lift their wings and mount up as eagles" (Isaiah 40:31).

CPSIA information can be obtained
at www.ICGtesting.com
Printed in the USA
BVHW080813310821
615687BV00007B/164

9 781098 028480